Ultrasound Examination of the Knee

Alternative method for diagnosis of meniscus lesions

Constantin Panow

I0494169

Printed by CreateSpace

Contents

"Ce qui se conçoit bien, s'énonce clairement, et les mots pour le dire viennent aisément."

(French: L'Art poétique – 1674- Nicolas Boileau-Despréaux.)

Disclaimer

The author and publisher decline responsibility about any injury or deleterious effect that could result from misinterpretation or wrong understanding and application of this text.

Key words

Meniscus lesion, knee, ultrasound, diagnosis, synovial plica, tendon fissure, osteoarthritis, tenosynovitis, joint sprain, collateral ligaments, neuropathic joint.

History of Ultrasound

Ultrasound has been poor man's modality since more than 50 years.

It attains exquisite definition, thanks to computer revolution, at turn of the century.

Able to visualize minute details and depict features far below 0.1 mm (0.004 inches) in size;

Modern machines become thus most performing technique in Radiology.

Only draw-back is contrast resolution;

Which in contradistinction with its space-counterpart;

Provides images of only average quality;

Unable to compete with other modalities?

Purpose of Title

More than 10 years after arrival on the market of those machines;

Their true potential has not yet been realized by medical community.

To this issue there are several explanations:

But the most prominent one, being training of specialists and learning curve.

If with MRI and scanner, an attendee is already well at ease after one single year of experience;

This is in no way the case with ultrasound.

Ugly images need years to become clear in one's mind;

And provide the right diagnosis.

The only difference between the States and Europe;

Is that we have a better pay back policy with insurance companies regarding this modality.

Bias of Economics

Still, in Switzerland, where I am working, reimbursement of ultrasound averages 160 bucks;

Which in comparison with MRI, more than 1000, is good value for money.

I try to make the best out of it, and as a consequence;

Would like to propose my experience to interested specialists;

As a valuable alternative to more expensive ones!

Aim

If I needed many years to finalize my aim;

Especially examining and diagnosing meniscus lesions with ultrasound;

Once I expose you the clear-cut of it;

You would be able to implement it in your daily practice within weeks.

Difficulty of Purpose

Why are radiologists unable to diagnose meniscus lesions with ultrasound?

Well, there are again several explanations to this difficulty.

The first, and most important is;

That they are trained the regular way!

Imagination is not only part of fiction;

As usual belief implies;

But, we are learning literature at first at school;

Not in order to be degraded by futile thinking;

But to imply it further in our daily work;

Once we are adults.

Philosophy

Philosophy is useless job only on the school bench.

Once you are living in the real world;

Things appear different!

A Matrix?

(Reference to the movie: The Matrix, with Keanu Reeves and Laurence Fishburne)

Imagination and philosophy get their true value and dimension.

Attitude

Pupils in my class in high school were memorizing for grades.

Me, I hated learning!

Understanding principles is always to be preferred to studying by heart!

(The Adventures of Scherlock Holmes, by Arthur Conan Doyle).

Here is the difference.

I am explaining you this, in order to make you grasp;

Why me, and not others, were able to master this problem.

And I know that many of my colleagues tried themselves at it.

Almost everybody, as far as I remember!

They would give up the trial after a few mistakes.

Me, I did not.

It is as simple as that.

And, if I succeed at it, you should be able too!

The main problem lies in the philosophy frame of this mystery.

As to practice, I am using this method on a regular basis since 8 years already.

Comparison with MRI

But, let us first envision another topic!

Why ultrasound?

I pretend not only ultrasound is a good alternative to MRI;

- *I mean it is the better one!*

Spatial resolution of modern machines exceeds by far the one of MRI;

Even in comparison with 3 Tesla machines;

Or even 6 Tesla ones?

No technique is able for the moment to document contrast resolution.

There is the problem of analysis of images.

Your brain needs to be trained appropriately at it.

Contrast resolution has to do with fine perception of details.

And this matter can be studied.

Very efficiently!

To elaborate this system I needed more than 3 years.

Once I expose you its details, you would be able to implement it in your armamentarium in a few weeks.

The other reason why MRI would never be as good as ultrasound:

Is that the meniscus of the knee is a superficial structure.

It lies only 1 mm (0.04 inches) under the epidermis in a skinny person.

This means, that with a 5-12 MHz probe;

Or 7-12 MHz one;

You are examining the meniscus of the knee with a frequency of 10 to 11 MHz.

This is High Resolution!

NO Way!

You would never be able to obtain such an image with MRI.

Well, there are guys who published similar pictures for wrist ligaments recently with high resolution. (MRI)

With Ultrasound it is just similar;

With a much lower interest rate on your bank account!

Let's go to the heart of it!

What is a meniscus?

Fibrocartilage!

It has a surface and an inner part.

It has fibers, which attach it to ligaments and capsule of the joint.

Its surface is smooth;

While it's inner part is soft.

What is the conclusion of these features on radiological pictures?

- Any interruption of surface should be considered abnormal!

Softer inner part means lesser elasticity!

Appearing less *echogenic* than surface.

As the meniscus is a triangular structure, pointing to the inner of the knee joint;

There would be an *artefact* projecting towards interior;

It can cause interruption of smooth surface of meniscus!

- If you angle the probe in an inappropriate way.

Now you start to envision, whence the misunderstanding;

Making colleagues unable to analyze this kind of images!

Issue Solved

The solution would be;

As with every ultrasound examination;

To angle your probe in a continuous way;

In order to analyze whether, what you see is real;

- *Or an artefact!*

Why me

And you would ask again:

- Why me, and not a better colleague?

Because I started to tackle this issue after I had already 10 years' experience with ultrasound!

The secret of English meadows:

Just mowing and watering!

For a few centuries.

(Old C. E. Eckersley- Essential English for Foreign Students, 1963)

Meniscus Fissure

Types of meniscus lesions of the knee:

- Most frequent one is *simple fissure.*

Can be on the lower or upper surface;

Would involve generally only a small segment of the structure:

That is, can be in the anterior, posterior horn, or in the middle (intermediate) part of the meniscus.

Posterior horn tears are typically encountered in women, who wear high heels.

Effect of beauty can thus be observed in lower extremities;

As a *hallux valgus,* or this kind of exquisite injury;

Which allows me to joke with some patients:
You forgot your better shoes at home today!

Distinguishing features of meniscus fissure and artefact:

Both interrupt smooth surface of meniscus.

As to the first one, it is tiny, cleft being less than 0.1 mm (0.004 inches).

The older the fissure, the more irregular its margins!

Scar tissue providing new surface to it, and hence difference in *echogenicity*.

The *artefact* is well defined only on one of its limits, usually proximal one.

Distal one appears sluggish, and badly delineated as such.

It is much wider, about as large as inner hypo-echogenic part of meniscus.

It disappears with different angling of your probe;

While a fissure remains constant!

Volumetric Representation

Not in space, as you are moving away and forward, in relation to your object of observation;

- Hence necessity to envision structures in space:

- *Which only use of the probe can teach you!*

Peripheral Tear

- Tear at the meniscus periphery:

This is a lesion of ligament fibers attachment.

Readily visible as simple interruption!

MRI is almost unable to depict such an injury.

Complex Lesions

- Bucket handle or free fragment.

Those are unusual lesions, which I see infrequently;

I do not observe more than 1% of such ones, as to whole number of cases.

They are easy to diagnose, as there is a gap between the two structures.

To distinguish bucket handle from free fragment;

It is sufficient to image continually the whole structure.

If there are two attachments to the rest of the meniscus, it is first;

If not- second possibility!

As to false negative rate of the method:

It is about 3 to 5 %, depending on age of the lesion.

Knees being examined on the first day of injury have negatives of almost 80%;

(It is the same logic, as with MRI).

What we see is not the lesion itself, but restructuring and healing process, which ensues.

In such cases it is sufficient to repeat ultrasound in one or two weeks,

A policy permitting to pinpoint all those meniscus lesions, which are escaping on first attempt!

An *old scar* is main differential of a fissure:

You would be able to obtain definite results;

And avoid confusion;

If you examine the same in several different positions;

Flexed, and extended, with different degrees of angling.

Knees of athletes, especially football players, can have many old lesions;

Opening of slit in meniscus, with bending of the joint;

Would allow you to coin the correct diagnosis!

Pain is, besides, absent in *scars*.

As to appearance on ultrasound:

They are slightly *hyper-echogenic*;

As any *scar tissue* wherever in the body;

Very old ones are just tiny lines within meniscus.

Sometimes sonographer is able to witness several meniscal scars in a football player.

Indirect sign

Indirect sign of meniscal tear is extra-synovial fluid collection of a few mm (0,04 inches) thickness along anterior surface of medial condyle for internal meniscus and lateral one for the external.

Baker cyst

Invariably companion of all meniscus lesions of the knee!

Physiology:

The Meniscus of knee joint is an *avascular* structure.

Only its periphery receives contribution of blood vessels.

Main structure is nourished like a sponge, by articular fluid.

It needs regular activity;

Especially walking;

Driving fluid out of it, when in load;

And sucking it in, while off- weight.

What this means, as a consequence in *pathology:*

Any lesion is provided with more nutriments by *synovial membrane*;

This lining produces fluid, and secretes all constituents needed for structural repair;

It also absorbs waste products.

- The knee has this particular escape phenomenon:

- The Baker cyst!

Which protects integrity of bone!

And allows to relieve overpressure from effusion inside the articulation:

 - To fill a *Baker cyst.*

- Located on medial side of popliteal fossa;

Between tendons of *semi-membranosus* muscle and *gastrocnemius*.

Sometimes just a slit;

Bigger in the evening, than in the morning;

Owing to activity.

It sometimes ruptures to fill subcutaneous tissue, and even muscular compartments of leg.

Common differential for deep venous thrombosis.

It is usually painful, or slightly sensitive, on pressure with the probe.

Which brings us to next subject in examination:

Importance of Anamnesis

As any other discipline in Medicine;

Radiology is not different!

Neither in its project;

Nor in its perspective of it;

First comes *diagnosis*;

Then *treatment;*

According to our philosophy of *Evidence Based Medicine!*

We start with *Anamnesis*;

And proceed to *Status*;

In Imaging, our tool is just different;

Being prolongation of our hands;

Phenomenology of injury is important as such;

Importance of Understanding

Denial of understandability of simple mechanics;

Being main provider of false diagnosis!

And with it wrong therapy;

Which is nothing else, than inefficiency!

Every structure examined thus;

Should be questioned in several ways, as to pertinence of observation;

Any objection, of any kind, should be examined carefully;

Under several aspects;

One of them depending on our machine;

Next to our perception of reality;

Then, the sensation of our patient!

And I joke frequently with them:

Main difference between my veterinarian colleagues and myself;

Is that my patients speak!

And, some even laugh.

Every single structural abnormality should be substantiated with adapted questioning:

First: - *Does it hurt?*

(When I am pressing on the suspected lesion with the probe).

Second: - I say at first: Forget about the first question!

(As some people get confused).

- *Is this the pain, for which you consult?*

This way of examination is important, because some lesions are very near to each other;

One knee can harbor several of them;

Some can be old;

Not relevant any longer!

Synovial plica

Located usually on the medial side of knee joint;

Less frequently on lateral aspect;

Can be observed beside *patellar* margin;

As a thickening in *synovial membrane.*

Manifests usually in early adolescence;

And late childhood;

As blocking in the knee joint;

Especially in flexion;

This allows diagnosis;

Snapping of this structure;

Over medial or lateral *femoral condyle*;

Can be observed in dynamic examination with ultrasound;

May be treated surgically;

But, most of the time is self- limited!

Improving after a few months or years;

Claimed to be inherited in etiology;

Not yet proved.

Fissures of tendons

Can be diagnosed accurately only with ultrasound!

(MRI would show them only if injected).

Once claimed in all locations as being inflammation!

Old view, similar to the one described in 19th century by Swiss surgeon Fritz de Quervain; (1895)

Nowadays practice with ultrasound shows;

That most of those so-called tendinitis;

Are in fact minute fissures of tendons!

True *teno-synovitis* does exist, but is much less common.

Inflammation of tendon and its synovia is bacterial in origin, similar to facet syndrome.

As to fissure of tendon, much more common;

Making up about 80-90% of cases in my practice;

It can be due to any *metabolic ailment*: (Metabolic syndrome)

Be it *diabetes mellitus*;

Hyper-lipidemia;

Or any illness, which taps in health of human organism;

Most quotation concerns *hyper-parathyroidism*!

In fact, in youngsters as in old age, most of the time, be it a tendon fissure, which is fresh, or does not heal after time appropriately, it is due to deficit in *essential fatty acids*:

Omega 3 and 6!

(Which are insufficient in quantity in everyday meals).

Correction of this main variable permits not only fissures to heal within 2-3 weeks, but also not to recur anymore.

Diagnosis

With ultrasound is simple:

A fissure is readily visible as such.

Most frequently in tendon of *popliteal muscle*;

Or tendon of *biceps femoris muscle*;

But may affect every single tendon around the knee.

Joint Sprain

Tearing of medial and lateral collateral ligaments:

Readily visible as more consistent gap in structures:

Occurring in 80% of cases at femoral attachment;

20% near tibial one;

And in 90% in anterior portion of those structures;

Only 10% in posterior part;

Most of the time, averaging 30% of fibers in extent of lesion.

Location depends on *lesional mechanism*:

Flexion and lateral rotation resulting in tear of anterior fibers of medial collateral ligament;

Extension, with same direction of movement of foot, - in lesion of posterior part of same;

You can infer from preceding the rest of this logic.

While amount of injured fibers depending on forces involved.

Fallacies in Anatomy

As to anatomy, specialists claiming complexity of lateral collateral ligament;

Which is supposed to be complex;

They have never examined the knee with ultrasound;

Otherwise they would know;

That, there is little difference between medial and lateral collateral ligament;

They are almost the same;

The *biceps femoris tendon*, attaching on head of *fibula*;

Being a separate element;

In ultrasound, as much as light-years away of what
they claim being same structure.

Then comes proximal *tibio-fibular joint*;

But this again, is another topic.

We are learning today Anatomy no more on dead
bodies, in decomposition;

But from living ones, and every day!

Joint effusion

In knee

Is readily visible in *supra-patellar recessus*, or
bursa;

Aim is showing, whether it is blood or else;

Difficult perspective, which is not always possible
with ultrasound;

In other body parts fresh blood being slightly *hyper-echogenic;*

And blood clot easy to define as such;

In synovial fluid mixing has particularity, that
clotting does not always occur.

Puncture is satisfactory method to prove nature of it.

MRI being able of better results in this respect!

Arthritis

Can be diagnosed with ultrasound, if there is thickening;

And/or *hyper-vascularity* on *Doppler* of *synovial membrane*;

Thick fluid in joint in this situation means pus!

Common bacteria, like Staphylococci provoke *erosions*;

- To be searched on all surfaces of bone;

And joint destruction, if left untreated:

- Ensues!

Lyme disease

Most common pathogen in Western Europe being Borreliosis:

As we live in its *Endemic zone*;

Tick bites go unrecognized in Geneva, where I practice;

Owing to different species of those insects;

Lyme's agent never destroys bone, in my experience;

But can cause prolonged ailment for several weeks, even months;

Arthritis is non-purulent;

And thus liquid analyzed in specialized labs is considered negative for bacterial infection;

(Germs do not grow on usual media!)

Treated early, in the first week, pain disappears in 3 days' time;

Which is to my opinion a valuable diagnostic feature and tool!

Anti-bodies for this disease being retrieved in laboratory only in 50% of cases!

(In my series).

Owing to many false negatives of this method.

Differential Diagnosis

Of such a radiological picture being:

Viral arthritis:

Parvovirus;

Arbo-viruses;

Some *Entero-viruses*, as well...

Gout and pseudo-gout

As known since centuries for first;

Those are metabolic illnesses!

Second is much more common;

Echogenicity of effusion depends on quantity of crystals present in fluid;

Deposits of *chondrocalcinosis* can be observed on all *chondral* surfaces;

Be it meniscus;

At first, as mere and minute points, which are *hyper-echogenic*;

Later, when readily visible with X-Rays;

As thin calcifications;

Should be searched for, appropriately, especially on cartilage of patella;

Gout causes *erosions*;

Which are *para-articular* in location;

And absent in most cases of *pseudo-gout;*

Some additional agent, concomitant with this one,
can also cause, this time, *articular erosions*;

In such a case;

As for instance, *Milwaukee shoulder*;

Destruction being a possible event;

A trained diagnostician should prompt labs check-up for disturbance of *phospho-calcic metabolism*;

As, for instance, in *primary hyper-parathyroidism*;

Or as secondary hyper-parathyroidism in chronic
renal insufficiency.

Osteoarthritis

Called Arthrosis in Europe:

Is well documented with X-Rays;

Every single feature of this pathology is also visible
with ultrasound;

Neuropathic Joint

One frequent confusion being a *neuropathic
articulation:*

Where disturbance in alignment occurs;

And is claimed by most specialists as being *osteoarthritis;*

As all other features are concordant!

Even old textbooks in Radiology fail to recognize this entity as such;

And describe *dis-alignment*, or *decentering* of articulation;

As one characteristic of this disease;

Nowadays diagnosis is easy;

As most of the time this is due to *Vitamin B12 deficiency*:

(Which cannot be diagnosed with labs dosage of this element!)

But may be shown with *homo-cysteine level* (for instance);

Elevated with deficit in Vitamin B12;

Which should be proved with a second dosage of *homo-cysteine* one month later;

After substitution with one single sub-cutaneous injection of Vitamin B12!

Early ultrasonic sign of neuropathic joint is thickening of collateral ligaments.

I hope you enjoyed this short text.

You can reach me at

http://www.thenopillshealthprospect.com

If you have any questions or comments, do not hesitate, write in my blog!